CANCER
PAIN
RELIEF

WORLD HEALTH ORGANIZATION
GENEVA
1986

First impression 1986
Reprinted 1987, 1988

ISBN 92 4 156100 9

TYPESET AND PRINTED IN SWITZERLAND
86/6766-Schüler-8000
86/7146-Schüler-6000 (R)
88/7659-Schüler-5000 (R)

Contents

Preface

In 1982, a WHO Consultation brought together in Milan, Italy, a group of experts in the management of cancer pain. These experts from the fields of anaesthesiology, neurology, neurosurgery, nursing, oncology, pharmacology, psychology, and surgery prepared a draft set of guidelines on the relief of cancer pain. The guidelines expressed the consensus that, using a limited number of drugs, pain relief was a realistic target for the majority of cancer patients throughout the world. Studies on the applicability and effectiveness of these guidelines have begun in a number of countries with different health care systems, under the direction of WHO and the WHO Collaborating Centre for Cancer Pain Relief at the National Cancer Institute, Milan.

The present book, which is based on the 1982 draft guidelines, was finalized following a WHO Meeting on the Comprehensive Management of Cancer Pain held in Geneva in December 1984; among the participants were experts in cancer pain management, in national and international legislation concerning the regulation of opioid drugs, in health care delivery, in health education, and in pharmaceutical research and manufacturing, as well as representatives of several international non-governmental organizations.

Introduction

Cancer pain relief is an important but neglected public health issue in developed and developing countries alike (*1*). Effective pain management, particularly in patients with advanced disease, is one of four priorities in a comprehensive WHO cancer programme, the others being primary prevention, early detection, and treatment of curable cancers.

It needs to be emphasized that relief is possible for the several million cancer patients who each day suffer unalleviated pain. Existing knowledge permits an approach to the problem that could be implemented on a worldwide basis. Analgesic drug therapy is an essential component of this approach (*2–4*); when used correctly, it is capable of controlling pain in more than 90% of patients (*5*).

Extent of the problem: prevalence of cancer pain

Cancer is a major world problem. Every year nearly 6 million new patients are diagnosed and more than 4 million die. This represents 10% of all deaths (*6*). Half of those who are diagnosed as having cancer and two-thirds of those who die of cancer are in developing countries. Pain is a common problem; an analysis of 32 published reviews revealed that 70% of patients with advanced cancer had pain as a major symptom (*7*), and of adults and children undergoing anticancer therapy, up to 50% experience pain (*8*). From the available data, it is not possible to give a precise figure for the worldwide prevalence of cancer pain because the total number of cancer patients receiving treatment is not known. A conservative estimate is that *every day* at least 3.5 million people are suffering from cancer pain, with or without satisfactory treatment.

A series of studies using verbal reports and rating scales indicate that pain is moderate to severe in about 50% of patients with pain, and very severe or excruciating in 30% (9). Several studies have demonstrated that the prevalence of pain increases as the disease progresses (8–10). Pain in patients with cancer frequently has multiple causes (8, 10). The common pain syndromes occurring in cancer patients have been described (11).

Numerous published reports indicate that cancer pain is often not treated adequately. An analysis of 11 reports, covering nearly 2000 patients in *developed* countries, suggests that 50–80% of patients did not have satisfactory relief (7). Many patients with advanced cancer and moderate to severe pain are not given sufficient analgesic medication to control their discomfort. They are restricted to a weak opioid[1] (e.g., codeine), or a stronger drug is given "on demand", instead of being given at appropriate regular intervals "by the clock". Estimates concerning relief of cancer pain in developing countries are not available. It seems certain, however, that most patients do not receive adequate therapy because of legal and other constraints on access to drugs, and notably to the strong opioids.

Nature of cancer pain

The definition of pain proposed by the International Association for the Study of Pain (12) may serve as a useful starting-point:

> "Pain is an unpleasant sensory and emotional experience associated with actual or potential tissue damage, or described in terms of such damage. Pain is always subjective. Each individual learns the application of the word through

---

[1] The word "opioid" is used in this report to refer to codeine, morphine, and related pain-relieving drugs.

experiences related to injury in early life. It is unquestionably a sensation in a part or parts of the body but it is also always unpleasant and therefore an emotional experience."

Several studies have evaluated the psychological factors that influence the severity of pain in patients with cancer (*13–15*). In patients with advanced disease, these factors are a major influence in determining the severity of the pain. A sense of hopelessness and the fear of impending death add to the total suffering of the patient and exacerbate the pain. Identification of both the physical and the non-physical components is essential to the provision of appropriate treatment. The concept of

Fig. 1. Influences modifying a patient's perception of pain

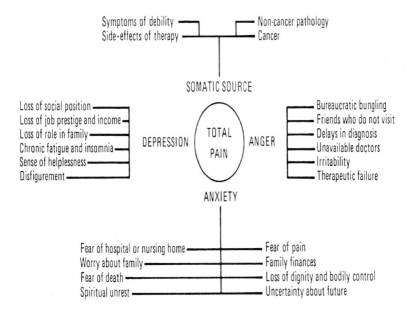

Symptoms of debility — Non-cancer pathology
Side-effects of therapy — Cancer

SOMATIC SOURCE

Loss of social position
Loss of job prestige and income
Loss of role in family
Chronic fatigue and insomnia
Sense of helplessness
Disfigurement

DEPRESSION

TOTAL PAIN

ANGER

Bureaucratic bungling
Friends who do not visit
Delays in diagnosis
Unavailable doctors
Irritability
Therapeutic failure

ANXIETY

Fear of hospital or nursing home
Worry about family
Fear of death
Spiritual unrest

Fear of pain
Family finances
Loss of dignity and bodily control
Uncertainty about future

[a] Reproduced from Twycross & Lack (3)

WHO 86746

"total pain" to encompass all relevant aspects is useful (Fig. 1). This includes the noxious physical stimulus and also psychological, spiritual, social, and financial factors (2, 3).

Recognition of the complex nature of cancer pain makes it easier to understand why some patients continue to experience intolerable pain even when given increasing amounts of analgesic medication. Unrelieved severe pain is often associated with a series of other symptoms, including disturbed sleep, reduced appetite, impaired concentration, irritability, and symptoms of a depressive nature.

It is important to stress that a clear distinction exists between patients with chronic non-malignant pain and patients with pain from progressive cancer. Extensive clinical experience has demonstrated that, while most cancer pain responds readily to established clinical treatments, this is not true of many non-malignant, chronic pain syndromes. Severe cancer pain commonly responds to strong opioid drugs, whereas this is not the case for most forms of non-malignant chronic pain. Where a patient's life expectancy is short, invasive techniques such as subarachnoid neurolysis and neuro-ablative surgery can be used more freely. The effects of these procedures, often unrepeatable, may last only a few months. While this may be sufficient for the terminally ill patient, it is clearly not suitable for those with a more normal life expectancy.

Cancer pain has been categorized according to a series of common pain syndromes and their pathophysiological mechanisms (3, 11). The first and most common cause of pain in cancer patients is that caused by tumour spread—for example, metastatic bone disease, nerve compression, and hollow-viscus and retroperitoneal involvement. The second group of pain syndromes, less frequent, is those associated with cancer therapy. These occur in the course, or as a result, of surgery, chemotherapy, or radiation therapy.

The physiological mechanisms of common cancer pain syndromes are not well understood. It is currently thought that a series of neuropharmacological and neurophysiological changes occur in bone, soft tissue, lymphatic vessels, blood vessels, nerves, and viscera, activating and sensitizing nociceptors and mechanoreceptors by mechanical (tumour compression) or chemical (metastases in bone) stimuli. Intermittent or continuous pain results. Analgesic drugs represent the first-line approach in controlling these kinds of pain. In some patients, tumour infiltration of a nerve or prolonged compression leads to partial damage to axons and nerve membranes, which become very sensitive to mechanical or chemical stimuli. The result is a superficial burning type of pain (dysaesthetic or deafferentation pain). In some patients the pain may also be stabbing (lancinating) in character. Deafferentation pain does not respond to opioids but is relieved to a variable extent by adjuvant drugs (16).

Present situation

The management of cancer pain has improved over the last 20 years. Numerous factors have contributed to the improvement, including better cancer diagnosis and treatment (4), a greater understanding of analgesic drug therapy, insistence of patients and their families that pain be better controlled, and a consensus that adequate symptom control and a good quality of life are particularly important in patients with advanced disease.

The development of the hospice movement in the United Kingdom heralded the continuing use of opioid analgesics administered orally to manage cancer pain (2, 3). The proliferation of modern hospices (palliative care units) and specialized pain relief centres in Canada, Italy, the United Kingdom, and the USA has provided supportive clinical experience (2, 3, 17), which has demonstrated that cancer pain can be treated effectively. The presence of a special centre also serves to raise the standard of cancer pain management in neighbouring hospitals (18, 19). The rapid increase in the number of professional health care workers who have become competent in cancer pain management suggests that such competence is readily transferable to a wide variety of situations (*19*). An example of this is the experience of the Saitama Cancer Centre in Japan (*5*), where 156 patients were treated in accordance with the draft guidelines prepared by a WHO consultation in 1982. Complete pain relief was reported by 87% of the patients, while "acceptable" relief was achieved in a further 9% and partial relief in the remaining 4% (*5*). These results indicate that professional and public expectations about the successful management of cancer pain can be raised considerably.

Drug therapy with non-opioid, opioid, and adjuvant drugs is the mainstay of such management. The effective use of these drugs requires an understanding of their pharmacological characteristics, the selection of a particular drug (or drugs) being geared to the needs of the individual patient (*2–4*). In a small minority of patients, neurolytic (*20–23*) and neurosurgical (*24, 25*) techniques are useful. It is possible, however, that their main benefit is that of procuring maximum relief more quickly. In one study, patients were treated either by drug therapy alone or by a combination of drugs and neurolytic procedures (*26*). After six weeks of supervised treatment, the degree of pain relief was comparable in the two groups.

The criteria for the use of neurolytic and neurosurgical procedures still need to be clarified. Moreover, these procedures are only rarely available as an option for the vast majority of patients. This is also true of behavioural approaches to pain control (*27–29*). In consequence, drug therapy is stressed in this book because of its crucial importance and widespread applicability. Several reviews of the use of oral and parenteral analgesics in the management of cancer pain offer practical guidance (*2, 30–32*). Medical groups and national committees have outlined approaches to drug therapy in the management of pain in advanced cancer (*33–38*). All have stressed the importance of providing adequate pain control and supportive care so that patients can enjoy a better quality of life and eventually die in comfort. These reports have also stressed the need to educate doctors and other professional health care workers in the use of opioid analgesics in the care of cancer patients (*33–38*).

Reasons for inadequate control of cancer pain

There are many reasons why not enough is done to control pain in cancer patients (*39–42*). Traditionally, the strong opioids have been used to manage acute severe pain, but their long-term use has been discouraged because of the possibility of the development of tolerance and physical and psychological dependence. *Tolerance* is a state in which increasing doses of the drug are needed to maintain the initial analgesic effect. *Physical dependence* is characterized by the onset of acute symptoms and signs of withdrawal if the use of the opioid is suddenly discontinued, or an opioid antagonist is administered. *Psychological dependence* is separate from both physical dependence and tolerance and is a concomitant behavioural pattern of drug abuse. It is characterized by a craving for the drug and an overwhelming concern with obtaining and using it. A misconception by doctors, nurses, and patients to the effect that physical dependence and psychological dependence are interchangeable terms has led to the under-use of opioid analgesics; lack of professional knowledge about their clinical pharmacological properties has further limited their effective use (*39, 40*).

In brief, the following are the major reasons for unsatisfactory management of cancer pain.

■ A widespread lack of recognition by health care professionals of the fact that established methods already exist for satisfactory cancer pain management.
■ A lack of concern by most national governments.
■ A lack of availability in many areas of the drugs essential for the relief of cancer pain.
■ Fears concerning "addiction" both in cancer patients and in the wider public if strong opioids are more readily available for medicinal purposes.
■ A lack of systematic education of medical students, doctors, nurses, and other health care workers about cancer pain management.

Comprehensive cancer pain management

A comprehensive approach to cancer pain management can be considered under three headings: pain assessment, therapeutic strategy, and continuing care.

Pain assessment

Assessment is a vital preliminary step toward the satisfactory control of cancer pain. It includes understanding not only the physical but also the psychological, spiritual, interpersonal, social, and financial components that make up the patient's "total pain". The responsibility for such an assessment lies primarily with the doctor. The main steps in the clinical assessment of cancer pain are described below. Ignoring them is a major cause of misdiagnosis and inappropriate management.

1 Believe the patient's complaint of pain.

2 Assess the severity of the patient's pain.

To assess the severity of the patient's pain, it is necessary to know the limitations on activity imposed by the pain, the number of hours of undisturbed sleep, and the degree of relief obtained from previous medication or pain relief procedures. Characterization of the patient's pain as mild, moderate, or severe provides a basis for appropriate drug therapy. Formal pain scales can be helpful but are not essential. Determination of the severity of the pain may be helped by asking the patient to relate the present pain to a past experience, for example, toothache, labour pains, postoperative pain, or muscle cramp.

3   Assess the psychological state of the patient.

Information about past illnesses, current level of anxiety and depression, suicidal thoughts, and the degree of functional incapacity helps to detect patients who may require more specific psychological support. Depression may occur in as many as 25% of cancer patients. Other common psychiatric syndromes are also seen in patients with cancer pain. Detecting these is an important part of the total evaluation of the patient.

4   Take a detailed history of the complaint of pain.

5   Perform a careful physical examination.

In assessing the patient with far-advanced cancer, a careful history and clinical examination may be all that is necessary to determine the cause of the pain and to facilitate the institution of appropriate treatment.

6   Order, and personally review, any necessary diagnostic investigations.

Investigations should be reserved for cases where there is doubt about the cause of pain, or where a decision about further anticancer treatment depends upon the precise localization of the disease. If anticancer therapy is not an option in patients with far-advanced disease, diagnostic studies play a less prominent role. Treatment with analgesic drugs, even while investigating the source of the pain, often markedly improves a patient's ability to participate in the necessary diagnostic procedures. There is no evidence to support the practice of withholding analgesics while the cause of the pain is being established. Pain control does not obscure the diagnosis of the cause.

7   Consider alternative methods of pain control during the initial evaluation.

Although drug therapy is the mainstay of cancer pain management, alternative methods are of considerable benefit for some forms of cancer pain. For exemple, patients with painful bone metastases generally obtain considerable, or even complete, relief through local palliative radiotherapy.

8 Assess the level of pain control after starting treatment

In patients in whom the response to therapy is less than expected, or in whom an exacerbation of pain occurs, it will be necessary to reassess the cause of the pain and the treatment strategy.

Therapeutic strategy

The therapeutic strategy proposed is described fully in Annex 1: Method for Relief of Cancer Pain. It relies upon the concurrent and sequential use of a series of treatment procedures (Fig. 2), which must be adapted to the needs of the individual patient. In many ways, this method is merely an outline. The details are likely to vary from country to country and from patient to patient. There is no specific reference to children. The general principles embodied are, however, commonly applied in paediatric cancer centres in the United Kingdom and the USA. The integration of the method into a more comprehensive programme of care for cancer patients is recommended. While complete relief of pain is not always possible, the method can be used to help all patients considerably. Previously intolerable pain can be eased to the extent that any remaining pain falls within the patient's ability to cope with it. In practice a sequence of specific aims is useful:

- increase the hours of pain-free sleep;
- relieve the pain when at rest;
- relieve pain on standing or during activity.

As shown in Fig. 2, the first approach includes anticancer treatments, if available and if appropriate. Symptomatic treatment measures should be used concurrently. These include

Fig. 2. Sequential approach to cancer pain management

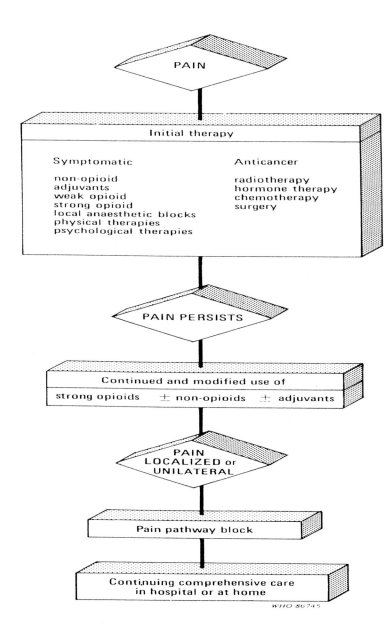

PAIN

Initial therapy

Symptomatic

non-opioid
adjuvants
weak opioid
strong opioid
local anaesthetic blocks
physical therapies
psychological therapies

Anticancer

radiotherapy
hormone therapy
chemotherapy
surgery

PAIN PERSISTS

Continued and modified use of

strong opioids ± non-opioids ± adjuvants

PAIN
LOCALIZED or
UNILATERAL

Pain pathway block

Continuing comprehensive care
in hospital or at home

WHO 86745

drug therapy, physical therapy, and psychological approaches. Temporary local anaesthetic blocks, such as trigger-point injections and regional anaesthesia, should be considered if available. If the pain is not adequately controlled, a strong opioid drug should be used, if necessary in combination with a non-opioid analgesic and adjuvants. When pain is localized to a dermatome or is unilateral, neurolytic and neurosurgical procedures may be of considerable benefit. These methods, however, are not widely available.

Drug therapy

The use of analgesic drugs is the mainstay of cancer pain management. When used correctly, analgesics are effective in a high percentage of patients. A three-step "analgesic ladder" is suggested (see diagram opposite). It is based on the premise that doctors and health care professionals should learn how to use a few drugs well. The three standard analgesics making up this ladder are aspirin, codeine, and morphine. Alternatives may be substituted, if necessary (see Annex 1, Table 3). These are proposed because the standard drugs are (*a*) not well tolerated by some patients, and (*b*) not available in all countries in an oral preparation.

In patients with mild pain, non-opioid drugs such as aspirin, paracetamol, or any of the non-steroidal anti-inflammatory drugs will be adequate. In patients with moderately severe pain, if non-opioids do not provide adequate relief when given on a regular basis, codeine or an alternative weak opioid should be prescribed. Non-opioid drugs, specifically the non-steroidal anti-inflammatory drugs, appear to act peripherally by inhibiting prostaglandin systems, whereas the opioids act centrally by binding to specific opioid receptors. Because of this difference, combinations of these two types of drug produce additive analgesic effects (*44, 45*), and are often used. In patients with severe pain, morphine—a strong opioid—is the drug of choice. It has a relatively short half-life, its pharmacokinetics are linear, and it is relatively easy to titrate the dose against the pain (*46–48*).

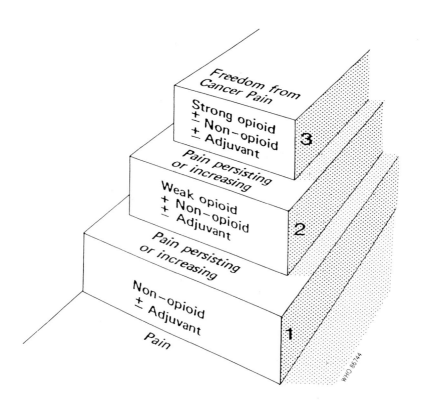

Adjuvant drugs are often needed in patients with pain secondary to nerve injury. There is evidence to suggest that they provide additive analgesic effects (49) and controlled studies demonstrate the analgesic efficacy of, for example, amitriptyline (16). Corticosteroids are commonly used in patients with cancer both as chemotherapeutic agents and as analgesics. Several studies have reported relief of pain by corticosteroids in patients with epidural spinal cord compression or infiltration of a nerve by the tumour, and also in metastatic bone disease (50, 51). Useful adjuvant drugs are listed in Annex 1, Table 3.

On the basis of considerable clinical experience and of controlled studies of analgesics, a series of important principles have been established:

1 *The dose of an analgesic should be determined on an individual basis.* The effective analgesic dose varies considerably from patient to patient. The right dose of an analgesic is that which gives adequate relief for a reasonable period of time, preferably four hours or more. The "recommended" or "maximum" doses described in standard textbooks are useful as starting doses only; more is often required. Unlike the doses of non-opioids, weak opioids, and mixed opioid agonist-antagonists, the doses of morphine and other strong opioids can be increased indefinitely. Published data indicate that it is rare for a patient to need more than 200 mg of morphine by mouth every four hours. Most patients need 30 mg or less (*2, 3*).

2 *The use of oral medication is preferable.* The patient taking medication orally is not restricted in activity by the route of administration. In contrast, the parenteral administration of a drug restricts the patient to either hospital or home and requires additional people to perform it. Data from hospices indicate that relatively few patients require injections to control their pain until the last two or three days of life (*2, 3*). For certain patients with intractable vomiting and pain, however, parenteral administration will be required. It is important to note that once the vomiting has been controlled it is generally possible to revert to oral administration.

3 *Insomnia must be treated vigorously.* Pain is often worse at night and prevents the patient from obtaining adequate sleep. This causes further debilitation. The use of a larger dose of morphine at bedtime, compared with the daytime, results in more prolonged relief of pain and better sleep.

4 *Side-effects must be treated systematically.* The common side-effects of the strong opioids–namely, constipation, nausea, and vomiting—must be monitored and treated with antiemetics and laxatives. Almost all patients receiving regular morphine require a laxative; about two-thirds need an antiemetic (*52*). Clinically important respiratory depression is, however, rare in conjunction with the chronic administration of strong opioids (*53*).

5   *Adjuvant drugs are necessary in certain patients.* An anti-
    depressant is indicated for patients who remain depressed
    despite improved pain control and for those with deafferen-
    tation pain (see page 11). An anxiolytic may be used for
    very anxious patients. Corticosteroids (*50, 51*), anticonvul-
    sants, and neuroleptic drugs also have a role to play in
    selected cases (see Annex 1).

6   *The patient's progress should be monitored carefully.* Cancer
    patients who are prescribed analgesics, whether opioid or
    non-opioid, need close supervision to achieve maximum
    comfort with minimal side-effects. An initial treatment
    review is sometimes necessary within hours, normally with-
    in one or two days, and always after the first week. Subse-
    quent follow-up will vary according to the specific needs
    of the patient. A new pain may develop. This calls for re-
    assessment, not just an increase in the current medication
    for pain, even though this may be an important initial step.

In summary, analgesic drug therapy in cancer patients with
pain usually achieves adequate pain relief. Sufficient data exist
to suggest that this particular approach can be readily transferred to non-specialist settings and generally applied in the
management of cancer patients suffering from unrelieved pain.

Other interventions

All pain is not equally responsive to analgesics. Neurolytic and
neurosurgical blocks may be necessary as a supplementary approach in a small number of cases. Although these techniques
provide an important respite from pain, the effect does not
last indefinitely. The main indication for these techniques is
activity-related pain associated with nerve compression. This
type of incident pain does not respond well to opioids. Neurolytic and neurosurgical blocks should be carried out only by
experienced specialists in a hospital or clinic (*4*).

The most useful neurolytic block is that of the coeliac axis
autonomic nerve plexus. This is reported as 60–80% effective
in patients with pain from cancer of the pancreas and other

epigastric neoplastic pain (23). Neurolytic blocks using phenol or alcohol are, however, relatively non-selective. Consequently, somatic nerve blocks may produce sensory and motor impairment or cause urinary and faecal dysfunction. The most useful neurosurgical procedure for cancer pain is percutaneous or open cordotomy (24, 54). Although this can be carried out by doctors other than neurosurgeons, it requires special training and regular application to maintain competence.

Continuing care

Pain control is but one part of a comprehensive approach to cancer patients. Continuing care is essential in order to ensure them the best possible quality of life. The National Hospice Organization in the United States of America has succinctly summarized the philosophy of continuing care: "[Continuing care] recognizes dying as a normal process... It neither hastens nor postpones death. [Continuing care] exists in the hope and belief, that through appropriate care and the promotion of a caring community sensitive to needs, patients and their families may be free to attain some degree of mental and spiritual preparation for death that is comfortable for them" (55).

The term "continuing care" is used in this book in a broader sense to include the care of a cancer patient from the initial medical assessment and diagnosis through evaluation and treatment, as well as during the final stages of disease, whether at home or in hospital. The availability of a caring professional health worker and, if possible, a caring team, is an essential component of such a programme.

The comprehensive approach to pain control advocated in these pages makes considerable physical demands and places great emotional stress on doctors, nurses, and other professional health workers taking care of cancer patients. Working within the framework of a team provides mutual support and encouragement. Teamwork is crucial for optimal care. The composition of the team will vary from patient to patient and from country to country. It is centred on the patient and includes the immediate family and others such as friends, neighbours, volunteers, doctors, nurses, therapists, social workers, psychologists and priests, etc. The team is collectively concerned with the total wellbeing of the patient and patient's family—physically, psychologically, spiritually, socially, and financially. In this situation, individual roles may overlap or even merge.

The major goals of continuing care are:

- Relief for the patient from pain and other distressing symptoms;
- Psychological care for the patient;
- A support system to help patients live as actively as possible in the face of impending death;
- Psychological care for the patient's family during the illness and bereavement.

These goals have been developed by the modern hospice movement (2, 3) and are employed widely in continuing care programmes. For the patient with pain, a continuing care programme is necessary to allow satisfactory titration of the dose of opioids and to control side-effects and other symptoms. Continuing care also prevents the patient from becoming socially isolated.

Education and training

Professional health care workers

Several reports have described the lack of education of professional health care workers in the management of cancer pain (*4, 36, 39, 42*). Education is a priority for ensuring the effective implementation of a cancer pain relief programme. Education in the management of cancer pain can be transferred to, and incorporated into, medical care systems, as is evidenced by the success of the hospice movement in several countries (*2, 3*) and by other reports (*5*).

The "Method for Relief of Cancer Pain" in Annex 1 provides a basis for the effective control of cancer pain and needs to be made available for educational purposes in both developed and developing countries. It is encouraging to note that several leading medical societies and governments have issued reports on cancer pain in recent years (*33–38*). These reports strongly urge the implementation of programmes of cancer pain management based on current knowledge of drug therapy.

Information about the nature and assessment of cancer pain and about therapeutic strategies should form the basis of any educational programme in this area. The aims of such a programme should be:

- to make available a common core syllabus containing the essential aspects of the Method for Relief of Cancer Pain—and also additional material aimed more specifically at the needs of each professional group;
- to provide training programmes for health care workers in conjunction with existing professional certification boards and the faculties of universities, colleges, and training schools;

- to incorporate the management of cancer pain into nursing and medical school curricula.

To maximize support for these proposals, cancer pain management should be:

- included as a compulsory subject in courses leading to certification;
- accepted as a suitable subject for testing by examination boards;
- recognized by universities as an appropriate subject for study, dissertations, diplomas, and higher degrees;
- recognized as an appropriate subject for scholarships, fellowships, and grants by academic institutions and research-funding bodies.

Progress is more likely if steps are also taken to:

- amend or adapt existing national laws in countries where medical education is legally directed, and facilitate appropriate educational programmes for health care workers;
- encourage and help societies and institutions interested in professional education (e.g., the International Association for the Study of Pain, the International Union Against Cancer (UICC), the World Federation for Cancer Care, national and international medical associations, specialist associations, postgraduate medical colleges, and cancer societies and foundations) and sponsor relevant conferences, seminars, and meetings at the local, national, regional, and international levels;
- provide a comprehensive list of suitable instructional material on cancer pain and symptom control, and facilitate access to such material through existing health education systems;
- encourage the support of industry in educating health care professionals and the public in the available approaches to cancer pain management.

The public

There is a need to reassure the public that:

- Cancer is not always painful.
- Treatment exists for the relief of cancer pain.
- Drug therapy is the mainstay of cancer pain management.
- There is no need for patients to suffer prolonged intolerable cancer pain.
- Pain relief drugs can be taken for prolonged periods and will continue to provide adequate analgesia.
- Psychological dependence is not an issue when strong opioids are taken to relieve cancer pain.

Legislative factors and substance abuse

Systems regulating the distribution and prescription of opioid drugs were designed before the value of the oral use of opioid drugs for cancer pain management was recognized. These systems were developed to prevent the social misuse of strong opioids; there was no intention to prevent the use of opioids for pain relief in cancer.

International and national drug laws

Of 22 drugs commonly used for cancer pain relief, eight are covered by the 1961 Single Convention on Narcotic Drugs and one by the 1971 Convention on Psychotropic Substances (56). The principal object of these two conventions is to stop trade in, and use of, controlled drugs, except for medical and scientific purposes. The conventions are not intended to be an impediment to the use of necessary drugs for the relief of cancer pain. It is therefore important that, by complying with the conventions, national laws should not, at the same time, impede the use of these drugs in cancer patients. Some countries have gone beyond the minimal control measures laid down in the conventions. Some have established stringent controls, especially in relation to drug prescription and distribution.

In a survey on the availability of drugs for cancer pain relief in WHO Member States, information was requested on the constraints and impediments interfering with the access of patients to the drugs. Information obtained from 38 countries demonstrated considerable diversity in national legal approaches as regards both the range of health care personnel and the types of distribution outlet legally authorized to handle drugs. There were considerable variations also in national approaches to prescription requirements. The existence of import quotas for both codeine and morphine was one of the constraints on drug availability.

In trying to understand the factors influencing the availability of drugs, it became apparent that in some countries responsibility for dealing with opioids is insufficiently integrated at the national level. There appears to be a lack of coordination between drug regulatory agencies, drug inspectorates, ministries of health, and the various government bodies responsible for drug procurement, drug pricing, industry incentives, customs, and law enforcement. It was noted that discussions and exchanges of views between these government agencies and the medical profession and pharmaceutical industry were inadequate.

In many countries, no strong opioid is available for oral use; often, opioids of the mixed agonist—antagonist class (e.g., pentazocine or buprenorphine) are the only opioids widely available, as this class of drugs tends to be less strictly regulated than the opioid agonist class (i.e., morphine and related drugs). Yet it is the strong opioid agonists that are recognized as the drugs of choice for the control of severe pain. Along with differences in legislation and distribution, countries varied in the security measures they employed for drugs from the time of manufacture or importation up to the time the patient takes the drug. The following findings, based on the data available and a preliminary assessment of specific problem areas, are worthy of note:

1 The proliferation of national laws and/or administrative measures regulating the prescription and distribution of opioid drugs necessary for cancer pain relief has hindered access by patients to these drugs.

2 Complex security measures result in elaborate record-keeping systems. Consequently, in almost all countries only extremely limited quantities of drugs are prescribable at any one time.

3   There is a lack of flexibility in existing drug distribution systems that prevents a wider variety of professional health care workers from prescribing and/or distributing drugs for relief of cancer pain.

4   Internally imposed import and distribution quotas impede availability of drugs to patients.

Further studies at both the national and the international level are indicated. These would be helpful in order to:

■   elucidate the relationship between the existing national drugs laws and the availability of pain relief drugs to cancer patients in each country;
■   develop a check-list of the essential features of an ideal regulatory system for opioid drugs (57);
■   identify ways that would enable cancer patients to obtain analgesics in areas where there is a shortage of pharmacies and doctors;
■   explore the hypothesis that excessive drug controls impede creative research into the development of strong analgesics.

The risk of substance abuse

In advocating a Method for Relief of Cancer Pain (Annex 1), the possible adverse consequences need to be considered. The development of a cancer pain relief programme should not be in conflict with programmes developed to control substance abuse and illicit drug trafficking, and vice versa. Concern with illicit drug use and its social consequences has, however, curtailed the availability of opioid drugs to patients with cancer pain. It is necessary, therefore, to examine what has happened in countries where oral preparations of strong opioid analgesics have been made available for such patients.

In this respect, Sweden provides a good example. The oral use of strong opioids did not gain widespread acceptance in Sweden until recently because oral administration was considered less efficacious than parenteral administration. Now, however, the regular use of oral morphine is considered the mainstay of the management of chronic cancer pain when non-opioid and weak opioid analgesics fail. This is reflected in the increase in the use of oral preparations of morphine and methadone in Sweden; there was a 17-fold increase in the use of morphine and methadone preparations between 1975 and 1982 (58). The increased availability of strong opioids has allowed a greater number of cancer patients to be cared for at home. Equally important, there has been no associated increase in illicit drug use or diversion of drugs to established addicts.

It should also be noted that the Method for Relief of Cancer Pain described in Annex 1 is for patients with advanced disease for whom the likelihood of recovery is limited; the risk/benefit factors related to substance abuse are minimal in this situation. There is also good evidence to suggest that legitimately supplied drugs contribute only minimally to the illicit market. A programme to make opioid drugs available for patients with cancer pain appears to be both feasible and of limited risk.

There is, in fact, very little published information assessing physical dependence or drug abuse in patients who receive opioid analgesics for any type of painful chronic illness. The incidence of opioid addiction in some 40 000 hospitalized medical patients has been monitored in a prospective study (59). Among nearly 12 000 patients who received at least one strong opioid preparation, there were only four reasonably well-documented cases of addiction in patients who had no history of drug abuse. These data from a survey of a general inpatient population suggest that the medical use of strong opioids is rarely associated with the development of addiction.

A series of studies reporting the abuse of analgesics in patients with chronic illness found that abuse of non-opioid analgesics or weak combinations of opioids and non-opioids was more common than abuse of strong opioid analgesics (60–62). Several recent studies, which describe continuing opioid therapy in patients with pain of non-malignant origin, report that continuing use of opioids is not associated with substance abuse or psychological dependence (63, 64). These studies support the view that drug use alone is not the major factor in the development of psychological dependence, but that other medical, social, psychological, and economic factors play an important role. These conclusions are also supported by studies of United States military personnel addicted to strong opioids in Viet Nam (65). In this group, drug abuse was strongly dependent upon a series of factors including underlying personality, social environment, and economic issues.

There is evidence to suggest that patients receiving opioid analgesics on a continuing basis develop some degree of tolerance to the analgesic effect of these drugs (66). Physical dependence also occurs, as evidenced by the appearance of withdrawal symptoms following the administration of naloxone, and by reports of acute withdrawal symptoms in patients who stopped drug therapy abruptly after being subjected to pain-relieving neurolytic or neurosurgical procedures (67). However, in studies of patterns of drug use in cancer patients, it was found that progression of metastatic disease causing increasing severity of pain was a major factor as regards the need to increase analgesic dosage (67, 68). Reduction of drug intake was associated with specific therapy directed at the cause of the pain. In another study, an absence of drug overdose, substance abuse, and psychological dependence was noted (43). It should also be pointed out that tolerance develops at different rates to each of the opioid effects. Tolerance to respiratory depression develops rapidly in contrast to the slow development of tolerance to constipating effects, if indeed tolerance to the latter develops at all.

Tolerance is only rarely a practical problem when strong opioids are used orally in the manner recommended in the Method for Relief of Cancer Pain (Annex 1). Often the first sign of tolerance is the patient's report that the analgesic effect is not lasting as long as it did. Such a report often labels the patient as a clock-watcher and is mistaken by professsional health care workers for an early sign of psychological dependence. In a controlled study, a shift in the dose-response curve to the right was demonstrated in patients receiving morphine on a continuing basis when they were studied at intervals of two weeks (69).

Organizational aspects

There are enormous differences in the medical resources of different countries. The recommendations made here will need to be modified in the light of local conditions. The successful implementation of a cancer pain relief programme requires adequate numbers of health care workers and adequate supplies of drugs and equipment. Its success will depend to a large extent on the willingness of the government to facilitate the provision of these prerequisites.

Health services

Major hospitals with cancer units

Each cancer unit should have a pain team whose role may be advisory, therapeutic, or educational. This team will include representatives of some of the following disciplines: anaesthesia, internal medicine, neurosurgery, oncology, orthopaedics, psychiatry, nursing, and social work. Members of the team will advise about, or care for, patients while they are in hospital and also, if necessary, after their return home. A hospital with a cancer unit should be capable of providing all the major forms of treatment for cancer pain management—namely, drugs, radiotherapy, and nerve blocks. Highly specialized techniques such as percutaneous cordotomy may also be available at this level. If the nearest major hospital is too far from the patient's home, the district hospital should be able to provide facilities for the satisfactory management of cancer pain.

Health centres

Although the name varies from country to country, the common feature of health centres everywhere is that they serve as the focus for medical care in the community. Health centres should similarly be the focus for the management of cancer pain in patients at home; in practice, this means the vast majority of patients with cancer. Hospital care, whether as an outpatient or an inpatient, should be kept to the minimum necessary to establish and maintain an appropriate regimen for pain relief.

The basis of care in the community is continuing professional supervision. Pain management is not the responsibility of the doctor alone but of all the professional health care workers involved. These workers need to be trained to evaluate patients, to advise patients' families about the various aspects of care, to understand the principles underlying the use of drugs in pain management, and to be able to provide psychological support for both patients and families. Voluntary helpers, including neighbours, may need to be recruited to provide sufficient care for patients with few or no family members. Equally important is the referral of patients to the agencies that, in some countries, offer financial assistance to patients with advanced cancer.

Hospices

Hospices will continue to play an invaluable role in establishing higher public expectations and better comprehensive standards of care for patients with far-advanced disease (*2, 3*). Hospices also provide opportunities for the education and training of health care workers from other areas. Some have become centres for clinical research in pain and symptom control. Although the consensus is that the widespread establishment of hospices is not the best way to make progress, their potential should be fully utilized, where they exist.

The family

For the patient with advanced cancer at home, the burden of care falls mainly on the family. Members of the family should therefore be trained to select and prepare suitable meals, to administer analgesics orally as well as parenterally, and to deal with instructions for handling specific medical problems (e.g., the management of the patient with paraparesis or paraplegia and of the incontinent patient). A loss of income on the part of a family member due to his or her own illness or to having to limit working hours because of the illness of another family member creates an impossible burden for many families. Where possible, sufficient government support should be available to enable patients to die at home if they wish.

Communication

Good communication between professional health care workers, patients, and patients' families is essential. Without it, patients often experience unnecessary distress and management is more difficult. Patients and their families should be informed of any available practical and financial assistance. Adequate information should be given in clear language that is easily understood. Among the members of the team caring for the patient, intercommunication about treatment goals, plans, and progress is crucial.

Summary of main proposals

1 Each national government should consider instituting a cancer pain relief programme. The participating agencies should include government departments of health, drug regulation, education, and law enforcement; national associations for professional health care workers; and other cancer organizations. Attempts should be made to raise, or reallocate, funds for the implementation of cancer pain relief.

2 Governments should share their experiences in designing drug regulatory systems to ensure that, while adequately combating drug abuse, these systems do not prevent cancer patients with pain from receiving the drugs necessary for pain relief.

3 National regulatory and administrative practices regarding the distribution of oral opioid analgesics should be reviewed and, where necessary, revision should be considered.

4 Governments should encourage health care workers to report to the appropriate authorities any instance in which oral opioids are not available for cancer patients who need them.

5 The Method for Relief of Cancer Pain (Annex 1) should be evaluated by national cancer centres, with progressive dissemination to the community level.

6 In a manner commensurate with their level of training, all health care workers should be taught to assess cancer pain and to understand its management.

7 Research into the management of cancer pain should be encouraged, in ways appropriate to the needs of each country. Such research should include the evaluation of existing pain relief services and the effects of changes in drug regulation and professional education.

8 Undergraduate and postgraduate teaching and examination and certification systems for nurses, doctors, and other health care workers involved in the care of cancer patients should emphasize knowledge of pain control.

9 Advanced cancer patients with pain should be able to receive care in their own homes, should they so wish.

10 Family members should be given training in the home care of cancer patients with pain, through the existing community health care systems.

Conclusions

Each day there are 3.5 million people suffering from cancer pain, many without satisfactory treatment. Yet established clinical methods exist for the effective control of such pain. Drug therapy is the mainstay of cancer pain management; relatively small amounts of inexpensive drugs suffice in the great majority of cases. Of particular importance are oral preparations of opioid drugs, notably morphine. Unfortunately, oral opioid preparations are not yet generally available in either developed or developing countries.

A broad educational programme is needed to teach health care policy-makers, doctors, and other professional health care workers about cancer pain management. Information about what is possible should also be disseminated to cancer patients and their families. National drug legislation should be amended, if need be, to facilitate the provision of drugs for pain relief to cancer patients who need them.

References

1 STJERNSWÄRD, J. Cancer pain relief: an important global health issue. *The clinical journal of pain,* **1:** 95–97 (1985).

2 SAUNDERS, G.M. *The management of terminal illness.* London, Edward Arnold, 1985.

3 TWYCROSS, R.G. & LACK, S.A. *Symptom control in far advanced cancer: pain relief.* London, Pitman Books, 1983.

4 FOLEY, K.M. The treatment of cancer pain. *New England journal of medicine,* **313:** 84–95 (1985).

5 TAKEDA, F. Preliminary report from Japan on results of field testing of WHO draft interim guidelines for relief of cancer pain. *The pain clinic journal,* No. 2, 1986 (in press).

6 WORLD HEALTH ORGANIZATION. Cancer as a global problem. *Weekly epidemiological record,* **59:** 125–126 (1984).

7 BONICA, J.J. Treatment of cancer pain: current status and future needs. In: Fields, H.L. et al., ed. *Advances in pain research and therapy,* vol. 9. New York, Raven Press, 1985, pp. 589–616.

8 FOLEY, K.M. The management of pain of malignant origin. In: Tyler, H.R. & Dawson, D.M., ed. *Current neurology,* vol. 2. Boston, Houghton Mifflin, 1979, pp. 279–302.

9 DAUT, R.L. & CLEELAND C.S. The prevalence and severity of pain in cancer. *Cancer,* **50:** 1913–1918 (1982).

10 TWYCROSS, R.G. & FAIRFIELD, S. Pain in far advanced cancer. *Pain,* **14:** 303–310 (1982).

11 FOLEY, K.M. Pain syndromes in patients with cancer. In: Bonica, J.J. & Ventafridda, V., ed. *Advances in cancer research and therapy,* vol. 2. New York, Raven Press, 1979, pp. 59–75.

12 INTERNATIONAL ASSOCIATION FOR THE STUDY OF PAIN. Subcommittee on taxonomy of pain terms: a list with definitions and notes on usage. *Pain,* **6:** 249–252 (1979).

13 SPIEGAL, D. & BLOOM, J.R. Group therapy and hypnosis reduce metastatic breast carcinoma pain. *Psychosomatic medicine,* **45:** 333–339 (1983).

14 CLEELAND, C.S. The impact of pain on patients with cancer. *Cancer,* **54:** 26, 35–41 (1984).

15 BOND, M.R. Psychologic and emotional aspects of cancer pain. In: Bonica, J.J. & Ventafridda, V., ed. *Advances in pain research and therapy,* vol. 2. New York, Raven Press, 1979, pp. 81–88.

16 WATSON, C.P. ET AL. Amitriptyline vs. placebo in post-herpetic neuralgia. *Neurology,* **32:** 671– 673 (1982).

17 TWYCROSS, R.G. & VENTAFRIDDA, V. *The continuing care of terminal cancer patients.* Oxford, Pergamon, 1980.

18 PARKES, C.M. & PARKES, J. Hospice versus hospital care: re-evaluation after ten years as seen by surviving spouses. *Postgraduate medical journal,* **60:** 120–124 (1984).

19 KANE, R.L. ET AL. A randomized controlled trial of hospice care. *Lancet,* **1:** 890–894 (1984).

20 COUSINS, M.J. & BRIDENBOUGH, P.O. *Neural blockage*. Philadelphia, J.B. Lippincott, 1980.

21 ARNER, S. The role of nerve blocks in the treatment of cancer pain. *Acta anaesthesiologica Scandinavica,* **74** (suppl.): 104–108 (1982).

22 SWERDLOW, M. Spinal and peripheral neurolysis for managing Pancoast syndrome. In: Bonica, J.J. et al., ed. *Advances in pain relief and therapy,* vol. 4. New York, Raven Press, 1979, pp. 135–143.

23 MOORE, D.C. Role of nerve blocks with neurolytic solutions in visceral and perineal pain. In: Bonica, J.J. & Ventafridda, V., ed. *Advances in pain relief and therapy,* vol. 3. New York, Raven Press, 1979, pp. 593–605.

24 FRIEDBERG, S. Neurosurgical treatment of pain caused by cancer. *Medical clinics of North America,* **59:** 481–485 (1975).

25 MEYERSON, B.A. The role of neurosurgery in the treatment of cancer pain. *Acta anaesthesiologica Scandinavica ,* **74** (suppl.): 109–113 (1982).

26 VENTAFRIDDA, V. ET AL. Comprehensive treatment in cancer pain. In: Fields, H.L. et al., ed. *Advances in pain research and therapy,* vol. 9. New York, Raven Press, 1985, pp. 617–627.

27 TURK, D.C. ET AL. Application of biofeedback for the regulation of pain: a critical review. *Psychological bulletin,* **86:** 1322–1341 (1979).

28 BARBER, J. & GITELSON, J. Cancer pain: psychological management using hypnosis. *Cancer,* **30:** 130–135 (1980).

29 MUNRO, S. & MOUNT, B. Music therapy in palliative care. *Canadian Medical Association journal,* **119:** 1029–1034 (1978).

30 BEAVER, W.T. Management of cancer pain with parenteral medication. *Journal of the American Medical Association,* **244:** 2653–2657 (1980).

31 INTURRISI, C.E. & FOLEY, K.M. Narcotic analgesics in the management of pain. In: Kuhar, M. & Pasternak, G.W., ed. *Analgesics: neurochemical, behavioural and clinical perspectives.* New York, Raven Press, 1984, pp. 257–288.

32 RANE, A. ET AL. Pharmacological treatment of cancer pain with special reference to use of oral morphine. *Acta anaesthesiologica Scandinavica,* **74** (suppl.): 97–103, 1982.

33 Socialstyrelsens kungörelse om medikament till smärbehandling i terminalvard. *SOSFS (M),* No. 21, pp. 1–9 (1979).

34 *Medicinalstyrelsens instruktionsbrev. Direcktiv om terminalvard.* Helsinki, 1980 (NO/NR 3024/02/80).

35 ROSETTI, P., ed. *Douleur et cancer.* Genève, Médecine et Hygiène, 1982.

36 AMERICAN COLLEGE OF PHYSICIANS, HEALTH AND PUBLIC POLICY COMMITTEE. Drug therapy for severe chronic pain in terminal illness. *Annals of internal medicine,* **99:** 870–873 (1983).

37 *Questions and answers about pain control. A guide for people with cancer and their families.* New York, American Cancer Society, 1983.

38 *Pain. A monograph on the management of pain/Douleurs cancéreuses – une monographie sur la conduite à tenir vis-à-vis des douleurs.* Ottawa, Ministry of Health and Welfare/Ministry of Supply and Services, 1984.

39 MARKS, R.M. & SACHAR, E.J. Undertreatment of medical inpatients with narcotic analgesics. *Annals of internal medicine,* **78:** 173–181 (1973).

40 ANGELL, M. The quality of mercy. *New England journal of medicine,* **302:** 98–99 (1982).

References

41 CHARAP, A.D. The knowledge, attitudes and experience of medical personnel treating pain in the terminally ill. *Mount Sinai journal of medicine,* **45:** 561–580 (1978).

42 BONICA, J.J. Cancer pain. In: Bonica, J.J., ed. *Pain.* New York, Raven Press, 1980, pp. 335–362.

43 BUKBERG, J. ET AL. Depression in hospitalized cancer patients. *Psychosomatic medicine,* **46:** 199–212 (1984).

44 HOUDE, R.W. ET AL. Clinical management of pain. In: Steven, S., ed. *Analgesics.* New York, Academic Press, 1965, pp. 75–122.

45 BEAVER, W.T. Comparison of analgesic effects of morphine sulphate, hydroxyzine and their combination in patients with postoperative pain. In: Bonica, J.J. & Ventafridda, V., ed. *Advances in pain research and therapy,* vol. 1. New York, Raven Press, 1976, pp. 553–557.

46 SAWE, J. ET AL. Steady-state kinetics and analgesic effect of oral morphine in cancer patients. *European journal of clinical pharmacology,* **24:** 537–542 (1983).

47 WALSH, T.R. Controlled study of slow release morphine for chronic pain in advanced cancer. *Pain* (suppl. 2): S202 (1984).

48 TWYCROSS, R.G. Choice of strong analgesic in terminal cancer: diamorphine or morphine. *Pain,* **3:** 93–104 (1977).

49 FOLEY, K.M. Current controversies in the clinical use of narcotics and related analgesics. In: Foley, K.M., & Inturrisi, C.E., ed. *Advances in pain research and therapy,* vol. 9. New York, Raven Press, 1985, pp. 3–12.

50 HANKS, G.W. ET AL. Corticosteroids in terminal cancer – a prospective analysis of current practice. *Postgraduate medical journal,* **59:** 702–706 (1983).

51 SCHELL, H.W. The risk of adrenal corticosteroid therapy in far advanced cancer. *American journal of medical sciences,* **252:** 641–644 (1966).

52 HANKS, G.W. Antiemetics for terminal cancer patients. *Lancet,* **1:** 1410 (1982).

53 WALSH, T.D. ET AL. High-dose morphine and respiratory function in chronic cancer pain. *Pain* (suppl. 1): S39 (1981).

54 TAKEDA, F. Neurosurgical treatment of chronic pain. *Postgraduate medical journal,* **60:** 905–913 (1984).

55 NATIONAL HOSPICE ORGANIZATION. *Standards of hospice programme of care.* Virginia, McLean, 1979.

56 REXED, B. ET AL. *Guidelines for the control of narcotic and psychotropic substances. In the context of the international treaties.* Geneva, World Health Organization, 1984.

57 JAYASURIYA, D.C. *Regulation of pharmaceuticals in developing countries. Legal issues and approaches.* Geneva, World Health Organization, 1985.

58 AGENAS, I. ET AL. Analgetikaterapi for cancerpatienter. [Analgesic therapy for cancer patients.] *Lakartidningen,* **79:** 287–289 (1982).

59 PORTER, J. and JICK, H. Addiction rate in patients treated with narcotics. *New England journal of medicine,* **302:** 123 (1980).

60 MARUTA, T. ET AL. Drug abuse and dependency in patients with chronic pain. *Mayo Clinic proceedings,* **54:** 241–244 (1979).

61 TENNANT, F.S. & RAWSON, R.A. Outpatient treatment of prescription opioid dependence. *Archives of internal medicine,* **142:** 1845–1847 (1982).

62 TENNANT, F.S. & UELMAN, G.F. Narcotic maintenance for chronic pain: medical and legal guidelines. *Postgraduate medicine,* **73:** 81–94 (1983).

63 TAUB, A. Opioid analgesics in the treatment of chronic intractable pain of non-neoplastic origin. In: Kitahata, L.M. & Collins, J.G., ed. *Narcotic analgesics in anaesthesiology,* Baltimore, Williams and Wilkins, 1982, pp. 199–208.

64 PORTENOY, R. & FOLEY, K.M. The use of opiates in chronic non-malignant pain. *Pain* **25:** 171–186 (1986).

65 ROBINS, L.N. ET AL. How permanent was Vietnam drug addiction? *American journal of public health,* **64:** 38–43 (1974).

66 FOLEY, K.M. Pharmacologic approaches to cancer pain management. In: Fields, H.L. et al., ed. *Advances in pain research and therapy,* vol. 9. New York, Raven Press, 1985, pp. 629–653.

67 KANNER, R.M. & FOLEY, K.M. Patterns of narcotic drug use in cancer pain clinic. In: *Research development in drug and alcohol use.* New York, 1981, (Annals of the New York Academy of Sciences, vol. 362) pp. 162–172.

68 TWYCROSS, R.G. Clinical experience with diamorphine in advanced malignant disease. *International journal of clinical pharmacology, therapeutics and toxicology,* **9:** 184–198 (1974).

69 HOUDE, R.W. ET AL. Evaluation of analgesics in patients with cancer pain. In: Lasagna, L., ed. *International encyclopaedia of pharmacology and therapeutics. Section 6: Clinical pharmacology.* New York, Pergamon Press, 1966, pp. 59–99.

Annex 1

Method for Relief of Cancer Pain

Contents

Introduction

The following brief account explains the principles of evaluating cancer patients with pain and provides a simple outline for the use of pain relief drugs. It represents the consensus of a group of experts on cancer pain management (Annex 2).

Cancer patients at all stages of the disease need to have their pain controlled. Pain occurs in about one-third of patients receiving anticancer therapy, but in more than two-thirds of patients with advanced disease. The physical basis of cancer pain includes a variety of mechanisms. The psychological aspects include anxiety, fear, depression, and a sense of hopelessness. The aim of treatment is to relieve the pain so that the patient can function effectively. Sometimes relief is complete, particularly when the patient is at rest; at other times the patient continues to have discomfort, particularly on movement (incident pain).

Drug therapy is the mainstay of cancer pain management. Drugs are effective in a high percentage of patients, if used correctly—the right drug in the right dose at the right intervals. The drugs discussed here are those most commonly used in patients with cancer pain. While controlled single-dose studies have demonstrated the safety and efficacy of these drugs and certain combinations of them, evidence on their continuing use is based mainly on wide and well-documented clinical experience. Some of the drugs are not available in every country. Where this is the case, drugs in the same class and of comparable analgesic efficacy should be used instead.

Evaluation of pain in cancer patients

Before deciding on treatment, it is essential to determine the cause of the pain. It is necessary first to study the history and the characteristics of the pain, and to assess the physical and psychological state of the patient. A detailed history must be taken to discover the location and distribution of the pain, its quality and severity, whether it is continuous or intermittent,

Table 1   Pain syndromes

	Nature of pain	Possible associated symptoms
Bone		
vertebrae	dull aching pain in cervical, thoracic, or lumbo-sacral region with or without radicular symptoms	spinal cord pressure symptoms (weakness, numbness, bowel and bladder dysfunction)
skull	localized tenderness	cranial nerve dysfunction
	headache	intracranial extension with brain and/or brain-stem symptoms
pelvis	dull aching pain in sacrum or hips or pubis	extension may be associated with sacral plexus, motor, sensory or autonomic changes
long bones	pain localized to site of tumour, but may be referred	disuse atrophy of muscles
	if pathological fracture occurs, patient will have severe pain on movement	local swelling and tenderness
Nerve		
cranial or peripheral neuropathy	pain, numbness in distribution of peripheral nerve(s) involved	paraesthesia, hyperaesthesia, dysaesthesia
	dull aching, burning pain possibly with bouts of lancinating pain	motor involvement
		reflex changes
	this pain may be due to nociception, nerve pressure, or both	autonomic changes

Table 1 *(continued)*

	Nature of pain	Possible associated symptoms
Nerve (continued)		
plexopathy (brachial, lumbar, sacral)	referred nerve pain in a limb	autonomic changes
epidural spinal cord compression	pain localized to vertebral body, radicular and band-like	sensory, motor, or autonomic changes; ataxia
meningeal carcinomatosis	headache or back pain radiating into lower extremities	increased intracranial pressure and confusion
		sensory, motor, and autonomic deficits
Viscera		
hollow viscus (i) thoracic	dull aching pain referred to chest wall	dyspnoea, cough
(ii) abdominal	dull aching pain referred to abdominal wall	abdominal distension, colic
solid viscus	progressively severe pain, epigastrium or right or left paraspinal region	jaundice, if pancreas and/or liver involvement
Other		
soft-tissue invasion	pain at site of tumour swelling if at superficial site	will vary with site of tumour

and what factors exacerbate or relieve it. Information should also be obtained regarding motor weakness, sensory deficits, mobility, and visceral dysfunction.

A careful examination should then be carried out of the patient's general physical condition, of the painful area, and of the relevant parts of the nervous system. In particular, the doctor should differentiate between local and referred pain (e.g., in cases of visceral involvement), between peripheral nerve and plexus or spinal cord involvement, between somatic and deafferentation pain, and between continuous and incident pain. In advanced cancer, incident pain is often movement-precipitated pain. This is less easy to relieve than persistent pain. If the pain relates to a pathological fracture or to a distinct acute condition, treatment specific to these conditions should be considered. When appropriate and available, anti-cancer treatment by radiotherapy, chemotherapy, or surgery forms part of the initial approach.

The causes of pain can be grouped under the following headings: (1) pain caused by the cancer itself, which is by far the commonest; (2) pain caused by the treatment (e.g., chronic postoperative scar pain, post-chemotherapy stomatitis); (3) pain associated with debility (e.g., constipation, bedsores); and (4) pain unrelated to the cancer (e.g., myofascial pains, osteoarthritis).

Many patients with advanced cancer pain have more than one of these pains simultaneously. Sometimes there are multiple cancer-related pains, or there may be pain due to cancer together with pain resulting from treatment.

Pain caused by cancer may relate to: (1) the bones; (2) nerve compression; (3) extension into soft tissues; (4) visceral involvement; (5) raised intracranial pressure; and (6) muscle spasm (secondary to bone pain).

It is important to assess the patient's pain carefully, as the treatment is dependent on the cause. Table 1 shows the type of pain that occurs when the cancer involves different tissues and structures, detailing other symptoms that may also be present.

Treatment strategy

Cancer patients often have many fears and anxieties. Some become very depressed. Highly anxious or deeply depressed patients may need an appropriate psychotropic drug in addition to an analgesic. If this is not appreciated, the pain may remain intractable.

Some cancer pains are best treated with a combination of drug and non-drug measures. For example, radiation therapy, if available, should be considered in patients with metastatic bone pain, or pressure pain from localized cancer. Moreover, not all pain is equally responsive to analgesics. Pain caused by damage to a nerve or to the spinal cord is superficial and burning (dysaesthetic) in quality. It is called deafferentation pain and does not usually respond to ordinary analgesics. It is important to recognize this type of pain as it is often helped by an antidepressant drug. Deafferentation pain may be associated with intermittent stabbing or shooting pain, which will respond to an anticonvulsant drug. There may be associated neurological signs, with or without an area of numbness (hypoaesthesia) in the pain region. Patients with deafferentation pain usually have a mixed pattern of pain and, in the presence of multiple pains, it may be necessary to use antidepressants as well as anticonvulsants with analgesic drugs (Table 2).

Table 2 Types of pain and implications for treatment

Type of pain	Treatment
Somatic (nociceptive) muscle spasm	physical therapy diazepam non-opioid analgesics
tissue distortion	analgesics
nerve compression	analgesics corticosteroids nerve blocks
Deafferentation (nerve destruction)	antidepressants anticonvulsants
opioids corticosteroids nerve blocks cordotomy	if peripheral nerve lesion, occasionally useful if spinal cord lesion, of no benefit

Use of analgesics

While the nature and cause of the pain are being assessed, therapy should be started with an appropriate analgesic drug. A decision to use anticancer treatment methods does **not** preclude the concurrent use of analgesics. An appropriate drug should be selected and treatment started at once. The three main analgesics are aspirin, codeine, and morphine. It is necessary to be familiar with one or two alternatives for use in patients who cannot tolerate the standard preparation. It is sometimes necessary also to prescribe one or more of a number of adjuvant drugs (Table 3). Two key concepts underlying the use of analgesics in cancer pain management are "by the clock" and "by the ladder".

Table 3 A basic drug list

Category	Parent drug	Alternatives
Non-opioids	aspirin	paracetamol
Weak opioids	codeine	dextropropoxyphene
Strong opioids	morphine	methadone pethidine buprenorphine standardized opium hydromorphone levorphanol
Adjuvants anticonvulsants	carbamazepine	phenytoin
neuroleptics	prochlorperazine haloperidol	chlorpromazine
anxiolytics	diazepam hydroxyzine	
antidepressants	amitriptyline	
corticosteroids	prednisolone	dexamethasone

"By the clock"

Analgesics should be given on a regular basis "by the clock". The dose of an analgesic should be titrated against the patient's pain, being gradually increased until the patient is comfortable. The next dose is given before the effect of the previous one has fully worn off; in this way it is possible to relieve the pain continuously.

"By the ladder"

The sequential use of the drugs is shown in the diagram below. The first step should be to use a non-opioid drug. If, in the recommended dosage and frequency, this is not effective in relieving the pain, a drug in the weak opioid group should be added to the medication given. When a weak opioid drug in combination with a non-opioid drug fails to relieve the pain, a strong opioid should be used. Additional relief may be obtained by giving aspirin in addition to the opioid, especially in patients with bone pain. Adjuvant drugs should be added to the opioid and non-opioid drugs, if required for specific indications (see p. 19). Only one drug from each of the groups should be used at the same time. *If a drug ceases to be effective, do not switch to an alternative drug of similar strength, but prescribe a drug that is definitely stronger.*

Annex 1, Fig. 1. The analgesic ladder for cancer pain management

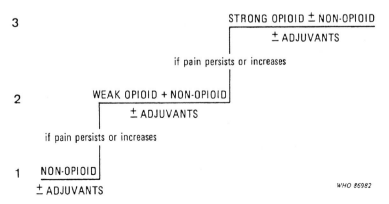

WHO 86982

Non-opioid analgesics

Aspirin and paracetamol are the commonly available non-opioid analgesics for the management of mild to moderate pain. These compounds have peripheral mechanisms of action. Aspirin is especially beneficial in metastatic bone pain, when a high local concentration of prostaglandins produced by the tumour cells is often present. Aspirin provides pain relief by blocking prostaglandin biosynthesis; it also has anti-inflammatory and antipyretic effects. In patients with bone pain who are intolerant of aspirin, one of the non-steroidal anti-inflammatory drugs commonly used in arthritic conditions should be considered. In patients with pain other than bone pain who are intolerant of aspirin, paracetamol is the alternative drug of choice. Non-opioid analgesics may also be effective in relieving pain caused by: (1) mechanical distension of periosteum; (2) mechanical compression of tendon, muscle, or subcutaneous tissue; and (3) mechanical compression of pleura or peritoneum.

Practical data regarding these drugs are given in Table 4.

Table 4 Non-opioid drugs

Drug	Suggested dosage	Side-effects
Aspirin	250–1000 mg every 4–6 hours	Gastrointestinal disturbance Fecal blood loss
Note:	The gastric side-effects may be reduced if aspirin is taken with milk, on a full stomach, or with antacids. The administration of more than 4 g/day serves only to increase the side-effects.	
Paracetamol	500–1000 mg every 4–6 hours	Liver toxicity
Note:	Use with caution in patients with liver damage. The total dose per day should be 2–6 g.	

Use of non-opioid analgesics

1   To avoid allergic phenomena, inquire whether the patient tolerates aspirin and aspirin-like compounds.

2   Non-opioid analgesics should be used regularly by the clock in order to avoid recurrence of pain.

3   An adequate amount of the drug should be administered. However, with the drugs in question, doses above those recommended will not give additional analgesia (see Table 4).

4   Non-opioid analgesics may be used alone or in combination with psychotropic or opioid drugs.

5   Side-effects (described below) should be looked out for; if they occur, change to an alternative non-opioid. If the side-effects are uncontrollable, consider administering a weak opioid.

Side-effects

1   *Gastrointestinal effects.* These are the most important side-effects. Aspirin may damage the gastric mucosa, causing erosive gastritis and gastric haemorrhage. Symptoms are heartburn, dyspepsia, nausea, and vomiting; objective signs are anaemia and blood loss in faeces. These may be exacerbated by concomitant cancer chemotherapy.

2   *Effects on haemostasis and coagulation.* Inhibition of platelet aggregation leads to prolongation of bleeding-time. In contrast to paracetamol, aspirin can have an irreversible effect on platelets, and the effect disappears only when new platelets are formed.

3   *Hypersensitivity.* The clinical manifestations of this relatively rare syndrome may develop within minutes of drug ingestion. They range from vasomotor rhinitis with profuse watery secretion, angioneurotic oedema, urticaria, and bronchial asthma to laryngeal oedema and broncho-

constriction, hypotension, shock, loss of consciousness, and complete vasomotor collapse. This reaction may occur in response to small amounts of aspirin.

Administration

Aspirin is normally administered in tablet form and should be taken after meals or with a glass of milk. Soluble preparations (e.g., dispersible and buffered aspirin) are available in some countries for patients with dysphagia; they are also less irritant to the stomach.

In most countries a range of aspirin-like drugs (nonsteroidal anti-inflammatory agents) is available. Some of these need to be taken only once or twice a day. Patients unable to take aspirin, but who would benefit from the use of an anti-inflammatory drug, may well tolerate one of these alternative preparations.

Paracetamol can be obtained as an elixir, a syrup, or a solution, but it is normally administered as a tablet.

When a non-opioid drug (with or without adjuvants) no longer controls the pain, a weak opioid analgesic should be combined with the non-opioid analgesic.

Weak opioid analgesics

The most important weak opioids are codeine and dextropropoxyphene. Codeine is to be preferred, but dextropropoxyphene is a useful alternative. These drugs are taken by mouth. Constipation is the main side-effect and can be prevented by the use of a laxative (e.g., senna). Nausea and vomiting also may occur. Physical dependence and tolerance may occur but are not a common problem with these drugs when used in pain management.

Codeine

An oral dose of 30 mg of codeine is approximately equivalent in analgesic effect to 650 mg of aspirin. When the two drugs are combined, the analgesic effect equals or exceeds that of 60 mg of codeine. Codeine may, of course, be used alone.

Suggested oral dosage (codeine phosphate in association with aspirin or paracetamol): 30–130 mg of codeine with 500 mg of paracetamol or 250–500 mg of aspirin every 4–6 hours.

Dextropropoxyphene

With repeated oral administration every 6 hours, a steady state is reached after 2–3 days. High doses occasionally produce central nervous system effects such as hallucination or confusion.

Suggested dosage: 50–100 mg of dextropropoxyphene in combination with 250–600 mg of aspirin or 500 mg of paracetamol present an anlgesic effect superior to that of each compound taken individually.

The drug is available as propoxyphene hydrochloride and propoxyphene napsylate; 100 mg of napsylate are equivalent to 65 mg of hydrochloride.

When the pain is no longer controlled by a weak opioid combined with aspirin or paracetamol (and, if necessary, an adjuvant), the patient should be started on a strong opioid.

Strong opioid analgesics

General considerations

Strong opioid analgesics are the mainstay of the therapy of moderate and severe cancer pain because they are simple to administer and, when properly used, they provide effective pain relief in most patients. These drugs are currently used on an empirical basis. The safe and rational use of opioid analgesics requires an understanding of their clinical pharmacology.

The use of strong opioid analgesics is associated with the development of physical dependence and tolerance. These are normal pharmacological responses to the continuing use of these drugs. Physical dependence is characterized by withdrawal symptoms if treatment is stopped abruptly. Tolerance is characterized by decreasing efficacy with repeated administration, and it may require an increase of the dose to maintain the analgesic effect. Physical dependence and tolerance do not limit the doctor's ability to use these drugs effectively.

Psychological dependence is a behavioural pattern characterized by craving for the drug and an overwhelming concern with obtaining it. Undue anxiety about psychological dependence ("addiction") has caused doctors and nurses to use opioid analgesics in inadequate doses. Wide clinical experience has shown that psychological dependence rarely, if ever, occurs in cancer patients receiving these drugs for chronic pain. In cancer patients, pain is an important symptom that can, and must, be treated.

It should also be emphasized that the continued use of oral morphine can be halted if the cause of pain is dealt with successfully by anticancer therapy (e.g., radiotherapy or chemotherapy). The dose should be decreased gradually, possibly over a period of three or more weeks. In this way withdrawal symptoms are avoided.

Many factors must be considered if these drugs are to be used effectively. These include: age of the patient, nutritional status, and extent of disease (in particular, involvement of the liver and the kidneys). In the elderly, lower initial doses should be used because of changes in the pharmacodynamics of the drugs and increased response. For malnourished patients, too, lower initial doses should be used, since malnutrition gives rise to changes in body composition and function. As the response of each patient varies, it is necessary to select the most appropriate drug and administer it in an individualized dose and by the simplest route. Oral administration is preferable, but in certain situations a drug might have to be administered sublingually, rectally, or parenterally.

The standard recommended dose must be adjusted according to individual need. This depends on the intensity of the pain, prior analgesic medication, and the distribution and availability of the drug in the body. The last-mentioned may be altered by intercurrent diseases, which may make it necessary to start with a lower initial dose and increase or decrease the dose according to the patient's needs.

Most strong opioid analgesics are metabolized primarily in the liver, and their elimination is therefore dependent on liver function. Liver dysfunction occurs with various tropical diseases. Involvement of the liver is not a contraindication to the use of opioids; in contrast to high doses of paracetamol and some of the adjuvant drugs, the opioid analgesics are not known to be hepatotoxic. However, care should be exercised when using them in patients with concomitant liver dysfunction. In patients with liver cirrhosis, the oral bioavailability (fraction of oral dose reaching the systemic circulation) has been shown to be increased for pethidine and for dextropropoxyphene. Concomitantly, the volume of blood cleared per unit time is decreased and the duration of action of the drugs is increased. This may lead to accentuation of the effects and the side-effects at comparatively low doses.

With few exceptions, the metabolites of most drugs are excreted by the kidneys. Therefore renal dysfunction leads to an accumulation of metabolites, some of which may produce toxic effects. Pethidine, for example, is metabolized to norpethidine, which may produce myoclonus and seizures at high concentrations. Its use is accordingly contraindicated in patients with severe renal dysfunction.

Some liver and kidney diseases are associated with low albumin levels, which may decrease the plasma-protein binding and hence increase sensitivity to analgesic drugs, including aspirin. Severe degrees of malnutrition may also alter the response to and the distribution and availability in the body of, these drugs. The lack of data on their effect on malnourished patients makes it necessary to exercise caution in their use. Malnutrition is not, however, a contraindication to their use.

Use of strong opioid analgesics

Morphine by mouth. Opioid analgesics must be administered in an acceptable form. The oral route is the best, because it spares the patient the discomfort of injections; it also maintains the patient's independence, since he or she does not have to rely on someone else for the next dose.

Morphine can be administered as a simple aqueous solution of morphine sulfate (or hydrochloride) in a range of strengths (e.g., 1 mg of morphine sulfate per ml to 20 mg per ml). An antimicrobial preservative is necessary, particularly in hotter climates. The taste is bitter, and some patients prefer to take the medicine with a drink to mask the taste. The solution should be stored in a dark bottle, which should be kept in a cool place and not exposed to direct sunlight. Morphine can also be made up in a syrup.

Sustained-release morphine tablets are available in some countries in strengths varying from 10 to 100 mg. The most widely available strength is 30 mg. These tablets normally need to be taken only every 12 hours. During the period of initial dose titration, a patient may need to take additional doses of sustained-release morphine or be supplied with aqueous morphine for "as required" use. Bioavailability and side effects are comparable with both immediate-release and sustained-release preparations.

The effective analgesic dose of morphine varies considerably and ranges from as little as 5 mg to more than 200 mg. In many patients, pain is satisfactorily controlled with doses of between 5 and 30 mg *every 4 hours.* However, the dosage varies greatly for different patients because of wide individual variations in the oral bioavailability of the drug; the appropriate dose is the one that works. The drug *must* be given by the clock and not only when the patient complains of pain. The use of morphine is dictated by intensity of pain and not by brevity of prognosis.

Instructions to patient. Emphasize the need for regular administration every 4 hours. The first and last doses of the day are "anchored" to the patient's waking and bedtimes. The best *additional* times during the day are generally 10h00, 14h00, and

18h00. With this schedule, there is an optimal balance between duration of analgesic effect and severity of side-effects. Ideally, the patient's drug regimen should be **written out in full** for the patient and his family to work from, including names of drugs, reason for use (e.g., "for pain," "for bowels"), dose (number of ml, number of tablets) and number of times per day. The patient should be warned about possible initial side-effects.

Choice of starting-dose (see also Table 5). The initial dose of morphine sulfate depends mainly on the patient's previous medication. For those who have previously received a weak opioid (e.g., codeine or dextropropoxyphene), a starting-dose of 5 mg may be adequate, though many require 10 mg and occasionally more.

If the patient is extremely somnolent after the first dose and is free of pain, the second dose should be *reduced* by 50%. If, after 24 hours on the medication, there is insufficient analgesia, the starting-dose should be increased by 50%. Meanwhile, the starting-dose can be repeated more frequently than 4-hourly to avoid excessive pain.

The patient must be reassessed after 24 and 72 hours, preferably by the doctor. If pain relief is not adequate or the drug being given causes unacceptable side-effects, another strong opioid drug should be tried. Sometimes the patient has a type of pain unresponsive to opioids, in which case non-drug measures (e.g., nerve blocks) should be considered, if available. Occasionally there is a marked psychological component to the

Table 5 Strong oral and sublingual opioid analgesics: starting-doses

Drug	Typical starting doses	
morphine	5–10 mg	by mouth
methadone	5–10 mg	
pethidine	50–100 mg	
buprenorphine	0.2–0.4 mg	sublingually

pain and an anxiolytic or antidepressant may be indicated. If no form of therapy provides relief, a search should be initiated for other factors that may be contributing to the patient's complaint of pain.

Night-time. The drug should be given through the night, or in a larger dose at bedtime, to sustain the plasma level of the drug within the effective range. With a 50% or 100% increase in the dose at bedtime, many patients do not need a further dose in the middle of the night.

Patients who require 60 mg or more of morphine usually need a middle-of-the-night dose to avoid waking in pain in the latter part of the night.

Control of unwanted effects

Nausea. If the patient has nausea when the treatment is started, prescribe an antiemetic concurrently, such as prochlorperazine (5–10 mg 8-hourly, increasing to 4-hourly), or metoclopramide (10 mg 8-hourly, increasing to 4-hourly). Haloperidol (1–2 mg daily) is a useful alternative.

If the patient is vomiting, the antiemetic will need to be given intramuscularly, possibly for up to 2 days. If the patient is free from nausea, it is generally advisable to issue a 4-day supply of an antiemetic to be used prophylactically or as required, in order to avoid initial nausea or vomiting.

Drowsiness. Warn the patient about initial drowsiness, but emphasize that this will clear up after 3–5 days on a constant dose.

Confusion. Warn older patients that they may become muddled at times during the first few days but should persevere.

Dizziness/unsteadiness. As for confusion.

Constipation. Almost all patients become constipated unless they have a colostomy or steatorrhoea. A laxative should be prescribed when morphine is started, and it should preferably be given at night. Dietary measures should also be taken if possible. *The control of constipation may be more difficult than the control of pain.*

For most patients, the regular use of senna counteracts the constipation. As in the case of morphine, the dose has to be titrated for each patient until a satisfactory result is achieved. Two tablets of standardized senna at bedtime is the usual starting-dose, increasing to 2 tablets 2–3 times a day, or more, if necessary. Some patients may require a second or alternative laxative. If the patient is severely constipated when an opioid is first prescribed, the use of suppositories or an enema is an important first step.

Morphine intolerance. In a minority of patients, there is persistent intermittent vomiting caused by delayed gastric emptying. A few patients experience marked persistent sedation. On rare occasions, a patient experiences psychotic symptoms, or symptoms relating to histamine release (pruritus, bronchoconstriction). These patients should be given an alternative strong opioid analgesic (see Table 5).

Alternative strong opioid analgesics

In most patients requiring a strong opioid, morphine is both efficacious and acceptable, and it is the drug of choice. If a patient appears to have persistent intolerance to morphine, an alternative that is chemically distinct should be used in the hope that this will not again cause the unwanted effect.

Methadone is a synthetic opioid analgesic with effects generally similar to those of morphine and is absorbed well whatever the route of administration. Given orally, it is about one-half as potent as it is when given by subcutaneous or intramuscular injection. Problems from its accumulation in the blood are likely to occur, especially in the debilitated and elderly. Maximum analgesia and side-effects are not achieved until after 4–14 days of use. Given in a single dose, methadone is marginally more potent than morphine but, in repeated doses, it is several times more potent. Its effective analgesic range is the same as that of morphine. It is generally longer-acting than morphine, useful analgesia lasting some 6–8 hours. Methadone, like morphine, has no obvious ceiling effect.

Greater care needs to be exercised in using methadone, as compared with morphine, particularly at first when the patient's response to it has not been fully evaluated. Extra care should be taken when psychotropic drugs are being administered concurrently.

Methadone should *not* be used

- in the elderly or demented,
- in those with confusional symptoms, or
- in patients with significant respiratory, hepatic, or renal failure

Rifampicin, an antituberculous antibiotic, speeds up methadone metabolism and may, on occasion, precipitate withdrawal symptoms.

Pethidine is a synthetic opioid analgesic. Its effects are generally similar to those of morphine. It also has atropine-like effects. It is about one-third as potent by mouth as by subcutaneous or intramuscular injection. It is about one-eighth as potent as morphine. It may not be as effective as morphine in relieving severe pain, but in higher doses it is considerably more effective than codeine. It is generally shorter-acting than morphine, useful analgesia lasting 3–4 hours.

Pethidine is *not* a complete alternative to morphine. It may need to be given every 3 hours in patients with severe cancer pain because of its shorter duration of action. Equally analgesic doses of pethidine and morphine produce a similar incidence of side-effects such as vomiting or depression of the respiratory centre.

With pethidine, the incidence of unwanted central nervous system (CNS) effects (i.e., tremor, twitching, agitation, and convulsions) increases considerably at doses above 200 mg 3-hourly. Pethidine should not be given to patients with impaired renal function because of the increased likelihood of CNS side-effects. Phenobarbital and chlorpromazine increase the toxicity of pethidine.

Buprenorphine, a strong opioid analgesic, is a representative of a group of opioid drugs called mixed agonist—antagonists. This class of drugs is a new development, and experience with them is more limited than with the older drugs. *They should not be used with other opioid analgesics* as they may reverse analgesia. Buprenorphine has a ceiling effect; it is *not* a complete alternative to morphine. Its morphine-like effects are greatest at a dose of about 1 mg intramuscularly. The onset of action occurs after about 30 minutes, and the peak effect comes after 3 hours (morphine, 1–2 hours). The duration of useful effect is some 6–9 hours (morphine, 4–5 hours). Most patients are satisfactorily controlled on an 8-hourly regimen. *The drug should be taken sublingually.*

The subjective and psychological effects are generally similar to those of morphine, but increasing the dosage leads to dysphoria, which is not the case with morphine. Compared with orally administered morphine, sublingual buprenorphine is some 60–80 times more potent. In patients whose pain is no longer controlled by buprenorphine, a change should be made to oral morphine sulfate. The initial starting-dose of morphine in this circumstance is determined by multiplying by 100 the previously administered total daily dose of buprenorphine. This total daily dose should be converted into a convenient 4-hourly regimen of morphine. Studies have shown that buprenorphine has a dependence potency less than that of codeine.

Other strong opioids

In some countries, some of the above opioids may not be available but other strong opioids can be obtained, most of which can take the place of oral morphine. The following should be satisfactory:

Standardized opium is virtually diluted morphine. The morphine content varies from country to country but usually represents 10% of the weight of opium powder. The doctor should determine the morphine content in his or her country. In some countries it is combined with aspirin in a fixed-dose tablet.

Hydromorphone is six times more potent than morphine. The duration of action is about 3 hours. The usual starting-dose will be 1 mg intramuscularly or 4–8 mg by mouth.

Levorphanol is five times more potent than oral morphine. It provides relief for 4–6 hours. Like methadone, it may accumulate in the blood and may produce sedation with repeated doses. The normal starting-dose is 1–2 mg intramuscularly or 2–4 mg by mouth.

Alternative routes for administering opioids

Rectal administration. Morphine may be given per rectum; this is as effective as by mouth. This route may be useful in patients who are vomiting or too ill to take oral medication. In some countries, suppositories are available in strengths ranging from 10 to 60 mg.

When suppositories are not available, it is possible to administer morphine by rectal enema, the dose being given in 10–20 ml of water. Opium and hydromorphone can also be given per rectum.

Subcutaneous or intramuscular injection. In patients unable to take oral or rectal opioid analgesics, the subcutaneous or intramuscular route should be used. Morphine, methadone, and buprenorphine may be given subcutaneously; pethidine must be given by deep intramuscular injection. The parenteral dose of morphine and pethidine will be about ⅓–½ of the previously satisfactory oral dose. In the case of methadone, the dose should be halved; with buprenorphine, the dose is unchanged.

When switching from the oral to a parenteral route, the patient's analgesic response should dictate the dose, as the recommendations given are based mainly on single-dose analgesic studies. Opium, hydromorphone, and levorphanol can also be administered parenterally.

Intravenous administration. Opioids may be given intravenously by either bolus injection or continuous infusion. It is, however, preferable to maintain the patient on oral drugs.

Epidural and intrathecal administration. These novel methods of administration have been developed to provide selective pain relief with minimal side-effects. They require special expertise for catheter placement and special equipment. Although effective, their role in cancer pain management remains controversial.

Adjuvant drugs

General considerations

The adjuvant drugs comprise a series of compounds of different chemical structure and are used for cancer pain management in one of two ways:

- to treat specific types of pain; or
- to ameliorate other symptoms that commonly occur in cancer patients.

Any attempt to formulate guidelines for the use of these drugs in cancer pain management must take the following considerations into account:

- The drugs were developed and released for clinical indications other than pain relief.
- Controlled studies of their use against cancer pain are lacking.
- The appropriate use of these drugs to enhance analgesia or to treat side-effects depends on careful assessment of the patient's symptoms and the clinical signs.
- Adjuvant drugs should not be prescribed routinely. The choice of drug is always dictated by the need of the in-

dividual patient. The drugs used to treat specific types of pain include anticonvulsants, antidepressants, and corticosteroids. The drugs used to ameliorate symptoms include neuroleptics, anxiolytics, and antidepressants (Table 6).

The concurrent use of two drugs that act on the central nervous system (e.g., morphine and a psychotropic drug, or two psychotropic drugs) is likely to produce a greater sedative effect in ill and malnourished cancer patients than in others. In

Table 6 Adjuvant drugs

	Analgesic effect	Anti-depressant effect	Anxiolytic effect	Muscle relaxant	Anti-emetic	Anti-con-fusional
Anticonvulsants						
carbamazepine	+ [a]					
phenytoin	+ [a]					
Psychotropic-drugs						
prochlorperazine			+		+	
chlorpromazine			+	(+)	+	
haloperidol			+		+	+
hydroxyzine	+		+		+	
diazepam			+	+		
amitriptyline	+ [b]	+	(+)			
Corticosteroids						
prednisolone	+ [c]	(+)				
dexamethasone	+ [c]	(+)				

[a] Often of benefit in lancinating (shooting, stabbing) pain.
[b] Often of benefit in dysaesthetic (superficial burning) pain.
[c] Often of use in nerve compression, spinal cord compression, raised intracranial pressure.

patients with cancer pain, the starting-doses of psychotropic drugs should usually be less than those commonly used for physically healthy patients.

Anticonvulsants

Phenytoin and carbamazepine are drugs whose mechanisms of action include the suppression of spontaneous neuronal firing. They have been used effectively in the management of specific neurological pain such as trigeminal neuralgia. In cancer, carbamazepine is useful in the management of the stabbing component of deafferentation pain.

The initial dose of *carbamazepine* is 100 mg a day, increasing by 100 mg every 3–4 days, to a maximum dose of 400 mg or occasionally 500–600 mg. The major side-effects include nausea, vomiting, ataxia, dizziness, lethargy, and confusion. These can be minimized by the slow upward titration of the dose and by close monitoring. Cancer patients are at a greater risk of developing leukopenia if they have recently received chemotherapy. The dose of *phenytoin* should commence at 100 mg a day and be increased gradually by increments of 25–50 mg to a total dose of not more than 250–300 mg per day. A steady state is achieved after 1–2 weeks. The side-effects are similar to those described for carbamazepine; they are usually mild and rarely interfere with therapy.

Neuroleptics

Chlorpromazine is not an analgesic and does not provide added analgesia when combined with an opioid drug. It does have antianxiety effects and may be useful in reducing anxiety that is exacerbating pain. It also has antiemetic and antipsychotic properties. Side-effects include hypotension, blurred vision, dry mouth, tachycardia, urinary retention, constipation, and extra-pyramidal effects. The dose is 10–25 mg orally every 4–8 hours.

Prochlorperazine is used as an antiemetic. The dose is 5–10 mg orally every 4–8 hours. Parenteral and suppository preparations are available.

Haloperidol is used most commonly for the management of acute psychosis and, in cancer, of patients in an agitated confusional state. It is a more potent antiemetic than chlorpromazine and is less sedative, with fewer anticholinergic and cardiovascular effects. A starting-dose of 1 mg by mouth once or twice a day is suggested. For the management of psychiatric symptoms, the doses are significantly higher—up to 10 mg 2–3 times a day.

Anxiolytics

Diazepam is commonly used to manage acute anxiety and panic. Anxiety is commonly seen in patients with pain, but this often diminishes once the pain is controlled. Diazepam does *not* provide additive analgesia when combined with an opioid drug. It is, however, useful in treating pain caused by muscle spasm. Side-effects include drowsiness, postural hypotension, and muscular hypotonia.

Dose: 5–10 mg of diazepam is the usual starting-dose. It can be given by mouth, per rectum or parenterally. Maintenance treatment ranges from 2–10 mg at bedtime up to 10 mg 2–3 times a day, depending on individual needs.

Hydroxyzine has anxiolytic, antihistaminic, antispasmodic, and antiemetic activity. When it is combined with morphine, additive analgesic effects occur. Side-effects include sedation, hyperexcitability, and multifocal myoclonus.

Dose: 10 mg three times a day to 25 mg 4-hourly, occasionally more.

Antidepressants

In cancer patients with pain, antidepressants are used to treat concurrent depression. Identifiable depression occurs in up to 25% of cancer patients. Antidepressants are also used to relieve the dysaesthetic pain of deafferentation. In this situation, antidepressants—notably amitriptyline—produce analgesic effects at doses below those used to treat depression. Amitriptyline also has a hypnotic effect, which helps to improve the patient's sleeping pattern.

The starting-dose of amitriptyline varies from 10 to 25 mg, given in a single dose at bedtime. A slow increase to 50–75 mg is usually associated with lessening of the deafferentation pain and improvement in sleep. In patients with major depression, daily doses of up to 150–200 mg may be required. Side-effects include dry mouth, constipation, urinary retention, light-headedness, and confusion. In rare instances, the drug may produce a hyperexcitable state. It is contraindicated in patients with glaucoma.

Corticosteroids

Corticosteroids may be used as adjuvant analgesics, for mood enhancement, and for appetite stimulation. They have anti-inflammatory properties and are useful in relieving pain associated with nerve compression, spinal cord compression, headache from raised intracranial pressure, and also bone pain. Both prednisolone and dexamethasone are effective; 1 mg of dexamethasone is equivalent to 7 mg of prednisolone.

The dose is dependent on the clinical situation. For nerve compression pain, 10 mg of prednisolone three times a day, or 4 mg of dexamethasone daily, should be prescribed, dropping to a lower maintenance dose after 7–10 days. Occasionally a higher dose is necessary to achieve significant benefit. With raised intracranial pressure, an initial dose of 4 mg of dexamethasone four times a day is appropriate. It may be possible to reduce this to a lower maintenance dose after 7–10 days. With cord compression, even higher doses have been used in some centres—up to 100 mg a day initially, tapering to 16 mg during radiation therapy.

Side-effects include oedema, dyspeptic symptoms, and, occasionally, gastrointestinal bleeding. Proximal myopathy, agitation, hypomania, and opportunistic infections may also occur. The incidence of gastrointestinal side-effects may be increased if corticosteroids are used in conjunction with aspirin-like drugs.

Summary

1 Cancer pain can, and must, be treated.

2 A thorough history should first be obtained and the patient examined carefully. Acute conditions that require specific treatment should be excluded.

3 Drugs usually give good relief, provided the right drug is administered in the right dose at the right intervals.

4 For persistent pain, the drugs should be taken regularly "by the clock" and *not* "as required".

5 For mild to moderate pain, the patient should be prescribed a non-opioid drug and the dose adjusted to the optimum level (see Table 4). If necessary, an adjuvant drug should also be used (p. 65).

6 If or when this treatment no longer relieves the pain, a weak opioid drug should be prescribed (see p. 54) in addition to the non-opioid drug, together with an adjuvant, if appropriate.

7 If and when these no longer relieve the pain, the patient should be prescribed a strong opioid, together with a non-opioid adjuvant drug, if appropriate (see p. 55).

8 The patient must be supervised as often as possible to ensure that treatment continues to match the pain and to minimize side-effects.

Annex 2

WHO meetings on cancer pain relief

WHO Meeting on Comprehensive Management of Cancer Pain[1]

(Geneva, 11–14 December 1984)

List of participants

Dr K. Bluglass, Department of General Practice Teaching and Research Unit, University of Birmingham Medical School, Birmingham, England

Dr J. Bonica, Department of Anesthesiology, University of Washington, Seattle, WA, USA

Dr L. Brasseur, Department of Anaesthesia and Resuscitation, Hôpital Paul Brousse, Villejuif, France

Dr E. C. Chidomere, Federal Ministry of Health, Yaba-Lagos, Nigeria

Dr L. J. de Souza (*Vice-Chairman*), Tata Memorial Hospital, Bombay, India

Sister P. Dittmer, Limburg/Lahn, Federal Republic of Germany

Dr I. Dunayevsky, Department of Anaesthesiology and Intensive Care, N. N. Petrov Research Institute of Oncology, Leningrad, USSR

Dr K. Foley (*Chairman*), Department of Neurology, Sloan-Kettering Cancer Center, New York, NY, USA

Dr L. Hemminki, Department of Public Health, University of Tampere, Tampere, Finland

[1] The World Health Organization gratefully acknowledges the financial support for this meeting provided by the Government of the Federal Republic of Germany.

Dr G. **Hundsdörfer,** Federal Ministry for Youth, Family and Health, Bonn, Federal Republic of Germany

Dr H. J. **Illiger,** Municipal Clinic, Oldenburg, Federal Republic of Germany

Dr D. **Jayasuriya** (*Vice Chairman*), Nawala, Sri Lanka

Dr **Liu Xu-Yi,** Institute for Cancer Research, Beijing, China

Dr M. **Martalete,** Department of Anaesthesia, Porto Alegre Hospital, Porto Alegre, Brazil

Dr M. **Max,** Education Committee, American Pain Society, Rockville, MD, USA

Dr L. G. **Paulo,** Division of Drugs, Manguinhos, Rio de Janeiro, Brazil

Dr I. D. G. **Richards,** Department of Community Medicine, Leeds, England

Dr M. **Swerdlow,** Manchester, England

Dr F. **Takeda,** Saitama Cancer Centre, Saitama, Japan

Dr R. **Twycross** (*Rapporteur*), The Churchill Hospital, Oxford, England

Dr F. **van Dam,** Antonie van Leeuwenhoekhuis, Netherlands Cancer Institute, Amsterdam, Netherlands

Dr C. W. **van Gruting,** Central Drugs Inspectorate, Ministry of Welfare, Health and Cultural Affairs, Leidschedam, Netherlands

Dr V. V. **Ventafridda,** WHO Collaborating Centre for Cancer Pain Relief, National Cancer Institute, Milan, Italy

Dr E. **Weber,** Clinical Pharmacological Institute, University Medical Clinic, Heidelberg, Federal Republic of Germany

Representatives of other organizations

Dr S. **Andersson,** International Association for the Study of Pain, Seattle, WA, USA

Miss M. C. **Cone,** International Federation of Pharmaceutical Manufacturers Associations, Geneva, Switzerland

Dr K. **Halnan,** World Federation of Cancer Care, London, England

Dr P. **Selby,** International Union Against Cancer, Geneva, Switzerland

World Health Organization

Dr M. **Abdelmoumène,** Office of Research Promotion and Development, WHO, Geneva, Switzerland

Dr M. G. **Dukes,** Pharmaceuticals and Drug Utilization, WHO Regional Office for Europe, Copenhagen, Denmark

Mr S. S. **Fluss,** Health Legislation, WHO, Geneva, Switzerland

Dr J. **Orley,** Division of Mental Health, WHO, Geneva, Switzerland

Dr D. **Schoenfeld,** WHO Collaborating Centre for Cancer Biostatistics Evaluation, Boston, MA, USA

Dr K. **Stanley,** Cancer, WHO, Geneva, Switzerland

Dr J. **Stjernswärd,** Cancer, WHO, Geneva, Switzerland (*Secretary*)

Dr M. **ten Ham,** Pharmaceuticals, WHO, Geneva, Switzerland

WHO Consultation[1]

(Milan, Italy, October 1982)

List of participants

Dr J. **Birkhan,** Rambam University Hospital, Haifa, Israel

Dr J. J. **Bonica,** International Association for the Study of Pain, Seattle, WA, USA

Dr P. B. **Desai,** Tata Memorial Centre, Parel, Bombay, India

Dr K. **Foley,** Department of Neurology, Sloan-Kettering Cancer Center, New York, NY, USA

Dr M. **Martelete,** Porto Alegre Hospital, Porto Alegre, Brazil

Dr A. **Rane,** Clinical Pharmacology, Huddinge Sjukhus, Stockholm, Sweden

Dr M. **Swerdlow,** Hope Hospital, Salford, England (*Chairman*)

Dr F. **Takeda,** Saitama Cancer Centre, Saitama, Japan

---

[1] The participants in this meeting prepared the draft guidelines on which the Method for Relief of Cancer Pain (Annex 1) is based. The assistance of the Floriani Foundation, Milan, in arranging this meeting is gratefully acknowledged.

Nurse F. R. Tiffany, Royal Marsden Hospital, London, England
Dr R. Twycross, The Churchill Hospital, Oxford, England
Dr V. V. Ventafridda, Division of Pain Therapy, National Cancer Institute and Floriani Foundation, Milan, Italy

World Health Organization

Dr F. van Dam, Antonie van Leeuwenhoekhuis, Netherlands Cancer Institute, Amsterdam, Netherlands (*Temporary Adviser*)
Dr R. Gelber, WHO Collaborating Centre for Cancer Biostatistics Evaluation, Boston, MA, USA
Dr K. Stanley, Cancer, WHO, Geneva, Switzerland
Dr J. Stjernswärd, Cancer, WHO, Geneva, Switzerland (*Secretary*)
Dr B. Wessen, WHO Collaborating Centre for Cancer Biostatistics Evaluation, Boston, MA, USA

Observer

Miss M. C. Cone, International Federation of Pharmaceutical Manufacturers Associations, Geneva, Switzerland

WHO publications may be obtained, direct or through booksellers, from:

ALGERIA : Entreprise nationale du Livre (ENAL), 3 bd Zirout Youcef, ALGIERS

ARGENTINA : Carlos Hirsch, SRL, Florida 165, Galerías Güemes, Escritorio 453/465, BUENOS AIRES

AUSTRALIA : Hunter Publications, 58A Gipps Street, COLLINGWOOD, VIC 3066.

AUSTRIA : Gerold & Co., Graben 31, 1011 VIENNA I

BAHRAIN : United Schools International, Arab Region Office, P.O. Box 726, BAHRAIN

BANGLADESH : The WHO Representative, G.P.O. Box 250, DHAKA 5

BELGIUM : *For books:* Office International de Librairie s.a., avenue Marnix 30, 1050 BRUSSELS. *For periodicals and subscriptions:* Office International des Périodiques, avenue Louise 485, 1050 BRUSSELS.

BHUTAN : *see* India, WHO Regional Office

BOTSWANA : Botsalo Books (Pty) Ltd., P.O. Box 1532, GABORONE

BRAZIL : Centro Latinoamericano de Informação em Ciencias de Saúde (BIREME), Organização Panamericana de Saúde, Sector de Publicações, C.P. 20381 - Rua Botucatu 862, 04023 SÃO PAULO, SP

BURMA : *see* India, WHO Regional Office

CAMEROON : Cameroon Book Centre, P.O. Box 123, South West Province, VICTORIA

CANADA : Canadian Public Health Association, 1335 Carling Avenue, Suite 210, OTTAWA, Ont. K1Z 8N8. (Tel: (613) 725–3769. Telex: 21–053–3841)

CHINA : China National Publications Import & Export Corporation, P.O. Box 88, BEIJING (PEKING)

DEMOCRATIC PEOPLE'S REPUBLIC OF KOREA : *see* India, WHO Regional Office

DENMARK : Munksgaard Export and Subscription Service, Nørre Søgade 35, 1370 COPENHAGEN K (Tel: + 45 1 12 85 70)

FIJI : The WHO Representative, P.O. Box 113, SUVA

FINLAND : Akateeminen Kirjakauppa, Keskuskatu 2, 00101 HELSINKI 10

FRANCE : Arnette, 2 rue Casimir-Delavigne, 75006 PARIS

GERMAN DEMOCRATIC REPUBLIC : Buchhaus Leipzig, Postfach 140, 701 LEIPZIG

GERMANY FEDERAL REPUBLIC OF : Govi-Verlag GmbH, Ginnheimerstrasse 20, Postfach 5360, 6236 ESCHBORN — Buch-handlung Alexander Horn, Kirchgasse 22, Postfach 3340, 6200 WIESBADEN

GREECE : G.C. Eleftheroudakis S.A., Librairie internationale, rue Nikis 4, 105-63 ATHENS

HONG KONG : Hong Kong Government Information Services, Publication (Sales) Office, Information Services Department, No. 1, Battery Path, Central, HONG KONG.

HUNGARY : Kultura, P.O.B. 149, BUDAPEST 62

ICELAND : Snaebjorn Jonsson & Co., Hafnarstraeti 9, P.O. Box 1131, IS-101 REYKJAVIK

INDIA : WHO Regional Office for South-East Asia, World Health House, Indraprastha Estate, Mahatma Gandhi Road, NEW DELHI 110002

IRAN (ISLAMIC REPUBLIC OF) : Iran University Press, 85 Park Avenue, P.O. Box 54/551, TEHERAN

IRELAND : TDC Publishers, 12 North Frederick Street, DUBLIN 1 (Tel: 744835–749677)

ISRAEL : Heiliger & Co., 3 Nathan Strauss Street, JERUSALEM 94227

ITALY : Edizioni Minerva Medica, Corso Bramante 83–85, 10126 TURIN; Via Lamarmora 3, 20100 MILAN; Via Spallanzani 9, 00161 ROME

JAPAN : Maruzen Co. Ltd., P.O. Box 5050, TOKYO International, 100–31

JORDAN : Jordan Book Centre Co. Ltd., University Street, P.O. Box 301 (Al-Jubeiha), AMMAN

KENYA : Text Book Centre Ltd, P.O. Box 47540, NAIROBI

KUWAIT : The Kuwait Bookshops Co. Ltd., Thunayan Al-Ghanem Bldg, P.O. Box 2942, KUWAIT

LAO PEOPLE'S DEMOCRATIC REPUBLIC : The WHO Representative, P.O. Box 343, VIENTIANE

LUXEMBOURG : Librairie du Centre, 49 bd Royal, LUXEMBOURG